ELEVATE

TO

GREAT

Brian Nunez

Ordering Information:
Quantity sales. Special discounts are available on quantity purchases by corporations, associations, and others.
Orders by U.S. trade bookstores and wholesalers. Please contact BRIAN NUNEZ via www.BrianNunez.com

Edited and Marketed By
DreamStarters University
www.DreamStartersUniversity.com

ACKNOWLEDGEMENTS

There are so many people in my life who have helped me throughout my journey. Without all of their support and the lessons I have learned from them, I wouldn't be where I am today.

First and foremost, I want to thank my number one partner in crime: my amazing superhero wife Parisa. Your unconditional love and support along with your passion to change the world inspires me every day. You gave me the greatest gift of all with our daughter Isabella who teaches me every day what patience, love, and empathy look like.

To my amazing mom, dad and stepdad who never missed a game and showed me the true meaning of family, sacrifice and hard work. You taught me the meaning of grit and the two most important things in life: attitude and effort. Thank you to my three, strong sisters Melissa, Lauren, and Kathryn who embody compassion, sympathy and care.

I want to thank all of the coaches throughout my entire lifetime who poured their expertise, passion, and faith into me. Specifically, Lance Fauria, Keith Allen, Todd Durkin, Greg Neiderlander and Grant Cardone for inspiring me to dream bigger and to hold higher standards for myself in my life. It is my duty and obligation to pay forward all that I've learned from those who have invested and believed in me.

I want to thank my amazing team, athletes and business partner Vijay Shah. You all embrace my crazy ideas, and I appreciate your patience and loyalty. I also want to acknowledge anyone who has ever worked for me and with me on the mission to coach people to live a fit, focused and free life.

Lastly, I want to thank Mike Fallat and his entire team at DreamStarters University for their help and support in bringing this book to life and inspiring me to share my story with the world.

I am humbled and honored to share my story and lessons to serve others just as so many people have served me. Thank you for taking the time to read this book and for wanting to ELEVATE your life to GREATNESS! You mean so much to me.

Table of Contents

"To be yourself in a world that is constantly trying to make you something else is the greatest accomplishment."

Ralph Waldo Emerson

Chapter 1

Elevate to Great

Is there anything worse than not having the freedom to be who you want to be and do what you were born to do? Living life *out of focus* might be a tragic close second, but freedom is the one thing we all seek. It took me many years of trial and error, mentorship, and learning through real world experiences before I was able to get focused, live a fit lifestyle, and find my own freedom. Once I did, life became an adventure that never seems to end. Nowadays, I help others do the same.

I grew up in a small town of about 80,000 people called Santa Maria, California. I don't remember a lot of my life until I was nine years old. That was when my parents got divorced. Everything before that point is kind of a blur for me. I don't remember much from when my parents were together. I guess that time of my life is just blocked off in my brain.

At nine years old, I woke up, and I started to become more aware of who I was. But my parents' divorce at that same time took a tough toll on me. I didn't understand it, and when I was young, I kept a lot of things to myself. I kept my emotions bottled up.

The divorce was not a clean, smooth process. It was very messy. I remember my parents fought a lot, and that was hard on me and my three sisters. We went from all living together, to bouncing around from one parent's house to the next, facing financial hardship, and not seeing each other every day. Although it wasn't easy, my parents always made sacrifices to try to give us the best opportunities to succeed.

My dad quit his job to try to save the marriage and focus on different things. I watched both of my parents struggle financially, but, regardless, they worked tirelessly to do everything they could to give me and my three sisters the opportunities they never had growing up. Witnessing bankruptcy and a messy divorce, I didn't really understand what these things meant at the time. I just knew that things were different for me than they were for my friends, and I was resentful of that.

I witnessed alcoholism as a child, and playing sports competitively helped me escape and distracted me from dealing with what was really going on inside of me emotionally. Even though I was well liked, I never wanted to show my true colors. I never wanted anybody to know who I really was. I acted very tough on the outside, but inside I was very insecure. I'm naturally a very introverted person.

I started playing football when I was five years old, and back then football culture was all about never showing any weakness or emotions and never acknowledging if you were scared or sad. This had a major influence on me. This tough mindset carried me through a lot of years, and it took me a long time to realize that allowing my true self to show through was not a weakness.

I constantly took my aggression and pain out through sports. Had I not been in sports, I don't know what I would have done with my life. I don't know where I would be now if I hadn't been a part of a team for many years. Who knows? I might have ended up in prison for taking my aggression out in an unhealthy way. There were so many things bottled up inside of me growing up, and sports were the only positive way I could express them.

I was never the biggest or fastest person on the team. But I was an insanely hard worker, and I had the determination needed to succeed. My upbringing helped me develop grit.

Nobody likes to go through hardship. Nobody likes to feel stuck in life, but I know the struggles I went through growing up made me into who I am today. They forced me to appreciate the journey of sacrifice, toughness and commitment I had to go through to become a better man.

I believe that understanding your roots and where you come from is so important for personal growth. A lot of times, however, people look at their past in the wrong way. They use their past as a justification for why they can't do something in their life.

They don't express any gratitude for all of the lessons they've learned in their lives and the people who have helped them along the way. When I was in my late teens and 20s, I had this kind of selfish mentality. I achieved a lot, and I had a lot of success in sports, but I was very unfulfilled.

It wasn't that I didn't like what I was doing, but I wasn't grateful for any of my success. In my mind, I was a victim, and everything I was doing was to block out my pain. It took me a long time to appreciate all of my life experience and see how it got me from point A to point B. I didn't have an understanding of myself, and I didn't have a connection to myself that I could appreciate.

Growing up, I saw the effects of what not exercising can do to your body. I saw what alcohol can do to people. These things showed me that I had to make a choice to go down an unhealthy path or a healthy one.

My biggest struggle growing up was that I was so emotionally dishonest with myself that I thought I had to live up to everyone else's expectations of me. I was so worried about maintaining the image of the popular jock and good-looking guy. This wasn't who I was, and I didn't care much about certain accomplishments other people told me were important.

I spent a lot of my early life trying to impress people, gain a certain status and maintain a certain label, but it was all draining. It was draining because I didn't know who I was. I knew who I was supposed to be in everyone else's eyes, but I didn't know myself. I would not wish this way of living on anyone. This is why my goal now as a fitness and overall life and business coach is to help people connect to their passion, purpose and greatest potential, so they can live a more fit, focused and free lifestyle.

My life experience has taught me that a connection to yourself is the number one thing you must have in order to live a happy, fulfilling life. Having a connection to yourself means you have a connection to what you're passionate about.

A connection to your purpose is what comes next. When you connect with your purpose, it gives you direction and a path to follow.

And, finally, a connection to your potential allows you to think bigger and imagine the possibilities of what your life could be like. A connection to your potential allows you to dream and create the next best chapter of your life.

If you don't give every part of your life the proper attention, then the changes you make to your life will not be long lasting and transformative. The purpose of this book is to help you discover the principles you can use to live your most fit, focused and free life. This book contains a game plan you can follow and action steps you can take to elevate your life from one phase to the next.

Throughout the book, you will find my personal stories mixed in with the lessons I teach all of my clients. I want you to know that everything I teach I've learned through personal experience, and I would never ask anyone to do anything I don't do myself. As you will learn later on in this book, one of my core values is practicing what I preach. In light of that, I hope you come away from this book with a sense of confidence, conviction and purpose that you have what it takes to *Elevate to Great*!

Chapter One

Lesson

"Personal Connection Leads to Greatness"

We all have a unique story to tell, but whatever your story is, you must own it. There is no right or wrong story. The only thing that matters is that you are authentic, honest and you don't compare *your* story with anyone else's. Your story is what makes you who you are. It's what makes you different, it's what makes you, YOU. Often times people feel the pressure to "one up" others, to have a worse or better story than someone else. What pain or pleasure feels like to one person may be completely harmless or boring to another. The point is, people shouldn't feel like they have to live up to society's (or another person's) standards when it comes to what is "acceptable" or what it means to live a great life.

Trying to please other people will only make you feel empty inside. I know this from first-hand experience. The number one way to feel disconnected from yourself is to not be your authentic self. This is what I struggled with for so many years, and this is why it is my passion to inspire people to share their truth and shine their light.

Your connection to *yourself* is the most important piece to living a happy, fulfilling life. Second is a connection to your *purpose*, and third is a connection to your *potential*. When you form all three of these connections properly, you are able to elevate your life to a place of success, happiness and ultimate fulfillment. I have realized that all of the struggles I faced growing up gave me strength. There were many things that I took for granted growing up, and I didn't focus my energy and attention on the positive. My lack of gratitude for my parents' hard work, support, and unconditional love is what made me realize later on in life that these are some of the most important qualities that a leader needs to have in order to serve and grow.

One of the biggest seeds to elevating to greatness in any and every aspect of your life is gratitude. The one thing I regret from my childhood is lacking gratitude for the sacrifices my family and friends made to support me. Whether you realize it or not, every person in your life has had some type of influence on you and the person you are becoming. The best way to shift into a positive state of mind and connect to yourself is to own your story and appreciate every single person along the way.

I have learned many valuable lessons that have helped me understand the importance of having a game plan for my life. This book is your game plan.

Game Changing Moves:

1. Be grateful for your roots!
2. What are the great qualities you learned from those who raised you?
3. Make a list of the great things you learned and who you learned them from.

(Please use the space below)

_____

_____

_____

_____

_____

_____

_____

_____

_____

_____

"A connection to yourself is the number one thing you must have in order to live a happy, fulfilling life."

#ElevatetoGreat
@CoachBrianNunez

Chapter 2

Happiness Comes from Within

When I graduated from high school, I went on to play Division 1 football. Many people doubted me, and they didn't believe I would make it to that high of a level, but it was a dream of mine. I was focused on attaining it, and I did.

But after my junior year, I didn't want to play football anymore. I decided I was done. I would finish out my four years of eligibility, however, I knew football wasn't something I wanted to pursue after college. My stepdad and my family were heavily invested in me continuing to play, but I knew it wasn't what I wanted to do.

I'll never forget my stepdad telling me, "If you keep playing football, I'll buy you whatever car you want. I'll buy you a BMW—literally, any car you want. I just want you to keep playing."

At the time, I was about 20 years old, and I didn't even know how to respond. In my head, I was just annoyed by the whole thing because I really didn't want to play sports anymore. I didn't understand what was going on underneath the surface of all this for my stepdad. The issue was that his value was placed in me, and not in his own life. As a parent now, I can see how that can happen. It can be tempting to put all of your energy into seeing your kids succeed and lose sight of your own success.

My stepdad was a hard-nosed, get the job done, bust your ass, kill-or-be-killed type of guy. However, he also had an amazing amount of passion for helping people. He helped me create an alter-ego that was hell-bent on crushing anything in its path on the football field. My stepdad put all of his chips in on trying to help me be great at sports. And when he did that, I believe he lost his connection to himself.

He did everything he could to help me succeed. He filmed all of my high school football games so he could coach me through what I needed to work on. I'll never forget Friday nights when I would get home after just playing a game, I'd walk in the house and my stepdad would already have the game film fired up and ready to go. Sometimes I'd have played a great game, but my stepdad would have a list of things I'd done wrong to show me on film, and he would push me to correct all of my mistakes.

He was obsessed with improving my game in a positive way, because he knew my potential. But I feel he lost himself along the way. I didn't realize for so many years that I took his leadership and love for granted, but when I decided I was done playing football, that was it for me, and that was it for my stepdad's dreams of me becoming the athlete he wanted me to be.

When I stopped playing sports after college, I decided I wanted to get away from everything and study abroad. I chose to go study in Australia on my own because I wanted to figure out who I was. I wanted to find myself. I didn't want to go with anybody I knew from school. I didn't want any kind of special treatment. I just wanted to start completely over.

My whole life, I'd been given special treatment because of who I was as an athlete. I had played the popularity game, and it worked for me, but I wasn't happy with it. I didn't like being treated like I was special just because I was good at doing something.

I wanted people to like me for me, but nobody knew who I really was. People liked me because of what I accomplished in sports, but nobody liked me for me. Even my relationships with my friends were just surface level.

I never felt like any of my friends had the same values as me. To be honest, I didn't even know what my values were back then, but I remember feeling like I wasn't on the same page with anyone. In fact, I felt like that for a long time.

My senior year of high school was one of the worst school years ever for me. I could not wait to be done with school and move on. I stopped hanging out with the group of friends I had, and I ate more lunches in a bathroom stall by myself than I can count.

You could say I was one of the cool kids in school, but I felt so alone and depressed my senior year. I was counting down the days until I could graduate because I felt so disconnected. I felt disconnected from myself, and I also felt disconnected from everyone else around me. I knew something was off, but I thought the change of environment when I got to college would put me back on track.

I thought that if I changed my environment, my feelings and mindset would change. A lot of people think this way. But this is not how things work. You can change the city you live in, the job you have, the friends you associate with and the amount of money you make, but unless you fix what's going on in your heart and in your head, nothing is going to change.

It's no surprise then that once I got to college, I started to feel the same as I had felt my senior year of high school. I still felt disconnected. I knew I wasn't living my life. I wasn't being myself. I was seeing chakra specialists and doctors trying to figure out what was going on with me, and I was hiding all of my struggles from all of my buddies.

As a D1 football player, the stigma was I needed to be even more of a bad ass, but my fuel was slowly running out. I knew if I kept trying to be who I was not, I was going to bust my skull open. I needed to rewire and get connected to myself and other people in a real way that wasn't based on anything but the real me. This is why I decided to give up sports after my senior season and go live in another country. I didn't know then that the changes I needed to make were all on the inside.

Chapter Two

Lesson

"The Road to Happiness Starts Internally"

It is common to think that you can change your environment and all of your problems will go away. But happiness and fulfillment don't come from outside circumstances. Happiness and fulfillment start on the *inside*. You have to face what's going on inside of you if you want to create positive change in your life. It doesn't matter what problem you are facing; the solution is always within.

Take a moment to reflect, and figure out what **the root problem** is that you are facing that is holding you back from elevating in one or more areas of your life. During different stages of your life, you will experience new challenges and obstacles. When I was in school, the biggest stress I had to worry about throughout the day was who was I going to eat lunch with or where could I find a place to be alone. All I wanted was to fit in and not feel like a loner. As I got older, I faced new sets of problems.

I believe that life drastically changes every 3 to 5 years. Since the day you were born, your life has changed drastically every 3-5 years. You've gone from being an infant to being a toddler, a toddler to a preschooler, a preschooler to a gradeschooler, and the list goes on. Every 3-5 years you are in a completely new environment with new challenges, new obstacles, new expectations, new rules, and new "successes." You may be fine in one phase of your journey but find yourself struggling in the next. In order to **elevate**, not transition, from one phase to the next, you must maintain a high sense of self-awareness and self-acceptance of who you are, what you stand for, and what makes you truly happy.

You can change your hardware, but until you can change and rewire your internal *software*, and face the battles and emotional viruses you've been going through, nothing will change. There will never be a time in your life where everyone loves you or everyone hates you. In life, there will always be people who like you and people who dislike you, but the only opinion that should matter is YOUR OWN. When you can enjoy spending quality time with yourself processing your own thoughts and emotions, you are one step closer to living free.

Game Changing Moves:

1. Make a list of the things and people that make you the happiest.
2. How much time do you spend doing those things and being with those people?
3. Commit to spending more time doing what makes you happy!

(Please use the space below)

_____

_____

_____

_____

_____

_____

_____

_____

_____

_____

"You can change the city you live in, the job you have, the friends you associate with and the amount of money you make, but unless you fix what's going on in your heart and in your head, nothing is going to change."

#ElevatetoGreat
@CoachBrianNunez

Chapter 3

Tragic Course Correction

I'll never forget when I got to Australia, I looked out the window in the room I was staying in, and I realized that I was completely alone. I had no friends there. I didn't even have acquaintances. Nobody knew who I was, and I was completely done with sports—something that had been a part of my life since I was five years old.

I was lost, but I realized that people were either going to love me for me, or they were going to hate me for me. It was scary, but it was what I wanted. I got a chance to challenge myself in an uncomfortable situation. I got the chance to meet new people and hang out with people as just a normal guy.

When my stay in Australia was over, I came back feeling good. I felt like I had figured some things out, and most of all I felt more connected to my real self and the friends I had made while I was away. I felt like they really appreciated me for me. I had accomplished my goal, and I was ready to keep the momentum going when I got back home.

But when I got back into my old surroundings and my old world, I was back to square one. All the people I had lost touch with came flooding back into my life. I was confused before I left for Australia, but now I was even more confused. I realized I hadn't really changed anything about myself. I had just changed the environment I was in.

As soon as my old social circle was a part of my life again, I got caught up in being the same old Brian that I didn't like—the same guy who was always trying to be Mr. Cool to everybody around him. I felt myself slipping back into disconnection from myself, and I started feeling very unfulfilled once again.

My mind screamed at me, "Hey! You're doing all the right things for all the wrong people again!" During this time, I struggled. Things were even worse than when I was playing sports because I didn't have any structure or team in my life anymore.

To cope, I didn't spend much time alone. I made myself busy by hanging out with my buddies, and I started partying a lot. I started dating and hooking up with girls all the time. I had shifted from trying to achieve success in the arena of sports to trying to achieve success with girls. While all of the guys around me thought I was living the good life, inside I knew I was not living the good life. I was living a very unfulfilled, very unpurposeful life.

Tony Robbins has a quote that really strikes me to my core. He says, "Achievement without fulfillment is the ultimate failure in life." I was doing things everyone around me thought were cool, but I knew I was failing miserably because I felt miserable. Slowly, I fazed myself out of the way I was living, and I started to focus on something positive. That positive thing for me was that I wanted to be a firefighter.

I was still in my early 20s, and I was kind of a dick. I had an attitude. I was ungrateful for the things that people did for me. I didn't appreciate all the sacrifices my family had made for me over the years. I didn't understand the investment they had made in me emotionally, financially or in any other way. I was just doing my thing, and I was selfish. This is why gratitude is such an important part of my life now.

Even though I was trying to focus on something positive and change things around, it was a slow process. I was still very much ego-driven. I was mainly focused on myself, and I wasn't thinking about other people. But life was about to throw me on a different course in the most unexpected way imaginable.

When I was 23 years old, I got a call from my sister very late at night. I had no clue why she would be calling me, but when I picked up, she told me through tears, "Brian, Jimmy is dead." Jimmy was my stepdad.

I couldn't believe what I was hearing. In my mind, I was thinking, "This isn't real. This cannot be real." So I asked my sister, "How did he die?"

And she told me, "He killed himself, Brian. He shot himself." I didn't even know how to process this information. It didn't make any sense to me at the time. My stepdad was just as much a father to me as my biological father, and him killing himself didn't even seem possible from what I knew about him.

In fact, my stepdad had a friend who killed himself in high school over a girl, and I remember him telling me the story about his friend and how he couldn't even believe how selfish his friend had been to take his own life. He had a very strong stance against suicide, and he had made it known to me.

On top of this, my stepdad was the person who taught me that it was either kill or be killed. For him, it was either you're going to kill me, or I'm going to kill you. But there was definitely no room in his thinking for killing himself.

After I had some time to process the news, I realized that my stepdad had been suffering from depression and alcoholism for a long time. When you combine those two deadly explosives together, something bad is going to happen at some point. The depression piece he hid from himself I believe by not connecting with himself at all. He invested so much of his life in me and my sisters. He lost the value of his own life somewhere in that process.

My stepdad's suicide was a wakeup call for me, because I realized that I was dealing with the same struggles that led him to do what he did. I was often depressed, and I also abused alcohol. Coming to this realization is what truly made me change the course of my life in a drastic way. I had to get back on the path I knew I was meant to be living, because I recognized that I was playing with fire.

Sometimes it takes tragedy in your life to force you back on to the correct path. I wish this wasn't the way it is, but I have experienced this reality firsthand. I believe the reason this is true is because when your heart breaks, you are forced to focus on it. You have to focus within to put your heart back together and come back stronger to pursue your purpose.

When you lose someone you love, it reminds you that your life isn't going to go on forever. Your time is limited on this earth. To make the most of it, you must connect with yourself and everyone around you in the most authentic way possible. The best way that I know to do this is through following your passion and using your unique gifts to serve others.

Chapter Three

Lesson

"Turn Your Struggles into Strengths"

Tragedy often inspires the biggest shifts in life. You don't often look at the core issues in your life until your heart is broken, and you have to look inward to repair it. When you lose someone you love, you learn to value the people in your life even more. We all know there will be tragedies that will happen in life. That is guaranteed! Life is short, and when we understand this reality as more than just a cliché, and we really start to live life with a sense of urgency and passion, we start to focus on what matters most.

Relationships are a huge part of life. Often times we hold grudges against people, don't communicate enough, or, as I regretfully did when I was younger, act like a complete jerk. When tragic things happen to someone important to you, they are final and there is nothing else you can do. You can't make that phone call to let that person know how much they mean to you. One of the worst feelings we can live with is the feeling of regret. Our own ego can hold us back from reaching out to people, apologizing, empathizing, or just checking in to see how someone is doing. Ego is usually the one thing that holds people back from achieving any type of greatness in their lives.

The one thing I will never get back in my life is the chance to tell my stepdad what he meant to me. I will never have that opportunity. Whatever relationship you have in your life that needs to be mended, remember that time is running out. Life is too short to not have clear, open, and honest communication with the people who mean the most to you.

Sharing your emotions with people and being honest with them allows you to not hold back any good or bad feelings. Make it a point to send daily text and video messages and to make phone calls to the people who mean the most to you. If your number was called tomorrow, would everyone in your life know how much they meant to you?

You learn a lot about yourself and your relationships when you start consistently communicating with people. You also learn that life is most fulfilling when you are doing what you're most passionate about and using your unique gifts to help other people.

Game Changing Moves:

1. What major tragedy in your life has helped shape who you are and how you think today?
2. How can you grow as a leader because of what you learned from and experienced in that tragedy?

(Please use the space below)

_____

_____

_____

_____

_____

_____

_____

_____

_____

_____

"Stop doing all the right things for all the wrong people!"

#ElevatetoGreat

@CoachBrianNunez

Chapter 4

Examine Your Roots

My transition into seeing the world differently took place much later in my life than I wish it would have, but all of my experiences have made me who I am today. All of my experiences have shifted my perspective in a way that I was able to connect fully with myself, and now I have the strength of that connection to draw on to help other people.

Ever since I was a kid, I have always wanted to help people. Of the few things I recall about my early childhood, I remember telling my mom that I wanted to start what I called a helping club when I was five years old. My mom didn't know what I meant when I told her this, so she asked me, "What are you going to help with? Are you going to help kids with their homework?" But that's not what I had in mind. I was focused on something else.

I told her, "No, that's not it. I want to help people—like if two adults are fighting, then I will step in, and I'll help them fix the situation." This was a pretty complex thought for a five year old to have, but I can only speculate now that it came from seeing my mom and dad fight all the time when I was growing up.

Somewhere in the back of my mind while I was struggling to connect with myself in high school and college, a part of me knew it was my destiny to help other people. I didn't know how I was going to do that exactly, but when I began to change my life following my stepdad's death, this is what I focused on figuring out.

I started doing personal training on the side while I was finishing up school and training to be an EMT and firefighter. Somewhere along the line, I felt the desire to shift into a more proactive role of helping other people. We need people who respond to emergencies like firefighters and police officers. They are absolutely critical.

But the other piece to the equation is that we also need people who help before an emergency happens. I felt drawn to helping other people on the front end, on the offensive side of things, because I wished I would have done more when I saw my stepdad suffering. I wished I would have had known that a simple conversation could have changed the direction of my stepdad's life.

But there were things that held me back from having that conversation. I was a young, punk ass kid in college, and I was focused mostly on myself. I didn't want to make myself vulnerable to other people. This was something I struggled with from a very young age.

Around the time my parents got divorced, I had to give this presentation at school that I was really excited about. It was a presentation about a Japanese puzzle, and I completely bombed when I got up to speak. The worst part wasn't that I embarrassed myself in front of the class. The worst part was that the teacher said to me in front of the whole class, "You didn't do this project right. Did you even research what you were talking about? Did you even try?"

This made me feel so small and insignificant, and all of my classmates were laughing at me. I left the front of the class completely ashamed of myself, and I went and sat down next to my friend. He looked over at me, and my face had turned white as a ghost as I sat there staring blankly.

He patted me on the back and said, "Hey, it's okay, man." But I couldn't accept any consolation or encouragement. Something in my mind clicked, and I decided right then and there that I was never going to speak up again. I decided I was never going to share my opinion with anyone, and I never wanted to be vulnerable with anyone again because I never wanted to feel as bad as I felt right then.

From that point on, I never wanted to speak in public. I failed most of the speeches I had to give in high school because I was so afraid of being judged. Of course, this is a long way from where I'm at now as a professional keynote speaker who speaks at conferences and events, but I struggled and had to overcome this fear that I lived with for a long time. The worst part was it affected more than just my ability to speak in public. It also affected my ability to express myself to other people in my personal life as well.

This root of shame and fear of embarrassment is something I had to dig out in order to become who I am today. There are so many things in my past that I had to overcome to live a fulfilling life, and my goal is to help people create the deepest level of change in their own lives possible.

This is why it's so important that you examine your roots. Doing this helps you understand who you are, where you came from, and even what sacrifices other people have made for you to get you to where you are now. You've got to create your path, and if you want to help a lot of people along the way, what's first and most important is you have to take care of you.

You may not like or agree with the things other people did to you or for you that brought you to where you are now, but you are here in this moment for a reason. The best attitude you can cultivate is gratitude about all of your experience, and the most important thing you can do is find the courage to change what's not working in your life. What you want for your life is on the other side of your fear.

Chapter Four

Lesson

"Learn from Your Past"

Everyone has had an experience in their past that has made a major impact on their present situation. There are always those one or two experiences, typically bad ones, that make people never want to do something again. I never would've imagined that I would be a professional coach and speaker, especially after having a huge fear of public speaking after my traumatizing childhood experience of being laughed at in front of my class.

This is why having a coach and surrounding yourself with positive and supportive people is valuable for you and your life. Sometimes we need to be pushed by other people to bring out the greatness inside of us. Sometimes we need someone to wake us up from believing a made up story that we've created in our mind throughout the years.

You have to listen to that feeling in your gut that is talking to you. That feeling of excited nerves misinterpreted as fear. That is not fear inside of you; that is the feeling of wanting to grow. It is your passion and energy wanting to be released! Once you know what is really holding you back, you can confront it head on.

39

I was so worried about being laughed at and what people thought about me for so many years. That is the opposite of living free. Your happiness cannot be determined by the applause of others. Your happiness must be driven by your own cause, and my cause has always been helping other people. However, for many years, I let my ego get in the way of that cause.

In order to succeed in helping others as a coach and professional speaker, I had to examine and overcome the root of my fear. What experiences have you had that are blocking you from living the life you want to live? What events in your past do you need to let go of in order to fully connect with yourself and live a life of purpose? You must cultivate gratitude for all of your experiences and find the courage to change. The life you were meant to live is on the other side of your fear.

Game Changing Moves:

1. Write down an experience in your past that has affected your confidence in your ability to grow.
2. What has this experience cost you in your life? (Trust, confidence, relationships, happiness, etc.)
3. What immediate, MASSIVE ACTION will you take to overcome fear and Elevate to Great?

(Please use the space below)

_____

_____

_____

_____

_____

_____

_____

_____

_____

_____

"The most important thing you can do is find the courage to change what's not working in your life."

#ElevatetoGreat
@CoachBrianNunez

Chapter 5

Playing a Whole New Game

When I graduated from college, I went all in on my life. I knew I had to figure out what I was going to do with my life for myself. I wanted to figure out exactly what it was going to take for me to live a free life.

It became my mission to discover myself. I went to Tony Robbins' conferences, and I started reading a lot of different self-development books. I hired coaches, talked to different professionals, and I started to embrace the importance of mindset when it comes to overall well-being.

As I studied all of this stuff more myself, a desire grew in me to help others with the same things I was learning. I had the background in sports that taught me a lot about fitness, but now I had the mindset piece I was lacking. I was missing that piece of the puzzle for a long time because I didn't see that true health begins with owning and embracing who you are.

Freedom comes from having conviction that you're on the right path, and then taking 100% responsibility and ownership of who you are, what you want, why you want it, and how you're going to get it with zero justification to anybody else but yourself. You have to convince yourself that you're worth all the effort, and you have to believe in yourself. It doesn't matter if other people agree with your path or if they don't like what you're doing. You've got to be yourself.

When I shifted from wanting to become a firefighter to wanting to focus on personal training, many people disagreed with my choice. I felt pressure from all different angles, including my parents, to make a different decision.

But I had realized that my desire to be a firefighter, while close to my intention of wanting to help other people, wasn't really what I wanted to do. My brother-in-law was a firefighter, and I thought I should do that too because it was a respectable job. But underneath all of my reasons for pursuing that path was me just being a copycat, and me going back to the same pattern of doing everything that everybody expected of me.

I had to decide to re-brainwash myself to believe that I could succeed as a personal trainer. Nobody thought being a personal trainer was going to be a lucrative or stable career for me. I had to fight against that and believe that it could be. I had to change my associations and the way I thought about it. The status quo didn't serve me, so I had to serve myself.

44

I remember in high school I had to do the same thing when my friends told me I was never going to play football at the next level. They told me I was too small, too slow, and overall not a good enough player to achieve the goal I had in mind of playing at the D1 level, but I didn't listen. I kept working hard, and I made my dream a reality.

Unfortunately, the truth is that the world is always trying to brainwash you. The world is always there making noise and trying to distract you from whatever you actually want to do. Other people will constantly try to get you to think like them, to fall in line and accept an average life.

People want you to have the same mentality as them no matter what. It doesn't matter who you surround yourself with. If you surround yourself with sick people, they're going to talk to you about being sick all day long and how the world is full of disease.

If you surround yourself with broke people, they're going to talk to you all the time about how the economy is bad. They're going to talk about how there are no opportunities out there for anyone to make a decent living.

But when you surround with people who say, "Dude, anything is freaking possible. Go after it," you start being able to take massive action. For me, I had to completely restructure the way I was thinking about things when I decided to become a personal trainer and go against the grain in my life once again.

I had to begin to believe that I could do what I wanted to do, and that I could help as many people as I wanted to help. I had to break outside of the rules of the game everyone around me wanted me to play by.

It's scary to do this, and it's not easy. When you leave for unchartered territory in your life, it's like you're playing a whole new game, and you're responsible for every outcome you experience. Nobody is holding your hand anymore or telling you what choices to make.

It's very hard to figure things out when you're no longer following a step-by-step plan. But the freedom that comes from living and playing the game by your own rules is what leads to ultimate success and happiness.

Chapter Five

Lesson

"Believe in Your Dream"

One rule I have for myself is not to surround myself with "should do" people. These are people who are always telling you what you "should do" based on what *they* think is best. The more you listen to these types of people, the more they will distract you from what you want and pull you outside of your lane.

Now, there *are* people who will give you great advice, but these are people who have already accomplished whatever it is you are trying to accomplish. They typically won't tell you what you "should do", rather they will tell you what you <u>need</u> to do. The point is that you need to be very selective with not only who you get your advice from, but also who you share your goals with. Not everyone will have the same vision, passion, risk tolerance or commitment you might have. This doesn't mean that those types of people are bad; it just means that you need to be more selective with who you get your advice from.

No matter what you want in your life, you have to believe it is possible. You have to believe in yourself and your ability to get the job done. The biggest thing that holds people back from achieving their goals is their limited belief in themselves and the possibility of being great.

Believe in what you want to accomplish, and surround yourself with other people who also believe in you. Nobody can hold your hand or tell you what choices to make in life, but when you accept 100% responsibility for your experience, it's like you're playing a whole new game. You are your only problem, and you are your only solution. You're free to make your own choices and decide how you want to live, and that's what leads to ultimate success and happiness.

Game Changing Moves:

1. If you knew you couldn't fail, what would you do?
2. Write down how you would feel not only pursuing your passion, but also having success in it!
3. Find a successful person in that space and learn as much as you can from them.

(Please use the space below)

_____

_____

_____

_____

_____

_____

_____

_____

_____

_____

_____

"Freedom comes from having conviction that you're on the right path, and then taking 100% responsibility and ownership of who you are, what you want, why you want it, and how you're going to get it with zero justification to anybody else but yourself."

#ElevatetoGreat
@CoachBrianNunez

Chapter 6

Play to Win

When I started my own business at 27 years old, I had no idea how much money I was going to make. I didn't know anything about business in general. I was not an educated guy in school; in fact, I was a 920 SAT score guy.

I basically had to resource my way through college, and what I mean by that is I had to surround myself with people who were way smarter than I was. I didn't care about school. I probably wouldn't have even gone to college if it wasn't to play football in the beginning. I was there to experience it, but I wasn't chasing any career dreams at the time.

I now run a successful multi seven-figure business, but I grew up going through two bankruptcies. I didn't know much about managing money because we never had much money. I also didn't know anybody who was a business owner except for my dad for a very short period of time.

My mind was never exposed to the rules of the game of business. But I knew I wanted to give myself a chance to succeed, and I knew I couldn't let the business failure statistics take me down without a fight. So I drew on what I did know about sports, and I thought to myself, "What can I do that will give me a chance to win in this game called business?"

When it comes to sports, winning is the only thing that matters. If you score more points than the other team, you win the game. If a game is on TV, and somebody walks in the room, the first question they ask is, "Who's winning?" They don't even have to understand the game being played to understand the answer to this question. They don't' have to know all the rules, because the question of who is winning is the only thing that really matters.

In sports, things are black and white. You're either winning, or you're losing. You don't get points for trying in any sport. In football, if you only make it to the one yard line, you don't get points. You have to take it all the way to the end zone, or you've failed.

But we don't approach life this way at all. In fact, the older we get, the less we try to win. We eliminate the scoreboard, and instead we just do things blindly. We mistake activity for achievement. We think to ourselves, "Well, I'm working 12-hour days, and I'm working my ass off 60 hours a week." But we forget to ask ourselves the more important questions.

We forget to ask ourselves what we're doing it all for. We forget to look at the results we're producing. Working a

12-hour day is not an accomplishment, and neither is working a two-hour day. Going to school and getting 10 different diplomas is not an accomplishment either, unless it helps you accomplish your mission.

Your mission will change over time, but you have to have one otherwise you will have no way to measure the results of what you're doing. You have to know what winning means to you.

For me, when I set out on the path to becoming a successful personal trainer, I had to create a scoreboard for myself. I had to create a way for me to know if I was accomplishing something or not. So the first financial goal in my career I set out to accomplish was to make enough money to buy a house.

I didn't even know what a mortgage was when I set this goal to buy my own house. I didn't know about insurance, or really much of anything about the adult world. I was never interested in that stuff in my early 20s. But my goal was to buy a house. If I could earn enough money to do that, to me that meant a win.

I set this goal in the year 2008 when the economy crashed. At the time, I heard people saying we were in a recession, but I didn't know what that meant. I kept hearing people talk about it, but I was too embarrassed to ever admit I didn't understand what they were talking about.

I was focused on training people. I'd hear stuff on the news about how things weren't looking good for people financially, but what I was hearing didn't line up with my life. I was in my lane, doing my thing, and I was making money. My ignorance was bliss, but the important thing was that I didn't get distracted by all the negative talk.

My priority was to give value to people, and I knew if I did that I would be rewarded. And I was. My business kept growing and growing until I finally had enough money to buy a house. When I bought my house, it gave me confidence and momentum because according to my scoreboard, I had won.

But then I had to reset the scoreboard and create a new goal. I wanted to grow the business at the health club I was working at, and because of the success I was having, they asked me to become the fitness director. At first, I didn't want to do it because I had a lot of freedom in my work, but it was a good enough offer that I decided to give it a shot.

I made it my mission to help the health club meet its goal every single month. But the energy level at the club was very low. It was like a funeral home of a gym. As fitness director, I knew we needed to revamp things. I knew we were never going to win by doing the same things over and over.

So I started a training class for a small group of people, and it did well. With that success, more resistance showed up. I was moving equipment around in the gym to better accommodate the training I was doing, and club members and other staff were getting pissed off.

I was ruffling everybody's feathers because I was changing things up. It got so bad that I decided if I couldn't do what I wanted to do inside the gym, then I'd take my training outside. And that's exactly what I did. I created my own training experience with no help from anybody else. My new goal was to get the people I was training profound results. If I could give them that, regardless of my methods, then to me that meant a win.

When you focus on what really matters, then you're focusing on the end result rather than the unimportant details. Focusing on winning is about focusing on the big picture. It's about putting your head down, and not getting frustrated when the results you want don't show up right away. Your goal is not to execute every single play perfectly, or to be the smartest guy on the field. Your goal is to win. Don't let what you don't know hold you back.

Chapter Six

Lesson

"Don't Mistake Activity for Achievement"

Too often people focus on the *activity* of trying to accomplish something rather than the metrics of accomplishing a goal, whether that is the number of hours worked, calls made, workouts done, or attempts performed. All of these things are extremely important actions to take in order to even give yourself a chance to win. The more you try, the more opportunities you have to win. Wayne Gretzky said it best, "You miss 100% of the shots you don't take." However, no matter how many shots you take at something, you will have to make some of those shots to actually win. *Doing* is simply not enough; you must do enough to put you in the best position to win in life.

Often times we hear that "success is trying your hardest." Although this sounds good and nice, it's not practical, real advice. There have been many times in my life where I've tried my hardest in sports and lost. Did that make me a winner? Not at all. I have lost in business while trying my hardest, working 80-hour weeks, spending little to no time with family, and still coming up short. I didn't get any wins for trying my hardest.

In life, there is no credit for "trying." You must win, and you can win. Does that mean you are going to win every time? Of course not. The only time I have really ever learned a valuable lesson is when I have lost. The losses expose weaknesses in you, your system, your process, your efficiency and your effectiveness. I would much rather take a loss and know what I need to work on than never take a shot at something and always wonder how I could have done.

Everything you do should have a scoreboard that tells you whether you're winning or losing. It's important to score everything objectively, from the relationships you have with people, to your fitness, to your career and goals.

In every aspect of life, you're playing to win. Don't let fear or what you don't know hold you back. You are a winner, and you were born to win. If someone else out there is accomplishing things you would like to accomplish, then it *is* possible. Now is your time to have laser focus and keep taking massive action until the job gets done. The job isn't done until the job gets done!

Game Changing Moves:

1. Create your own scoreboard! Is it pounds to lose, money to make, house to buy, etc.? Write down all of the wins you want to accomplish.

2. In what ways have you been mistaking activity for achievement? (Long hours worked, courses taken, seminars and conferences attended, etc.)

3. What are three things you will achieve this year?

(Please use the space below)

_____

_____

_____

_____

_____

_____

_____

_____

_____

_____

"Don't let what you don't know hold you back."

#ElevatetoGreat
@CoachBrianNunez

Chapter 7

Dumpster Dive Your Way to Success

When I was 11 years old, I started digging through dumpsters. I was living in an apartment complex with my mom and sisters after my parents divorced, and neither of them had much money, so I never had much either. My friends got money for doing chores around the house and things like that, so they were always able to buy little things they wanted like candy.

It always bothered me to see them with candy when I didn't have any. I've always had a sweet tooth, and my favorite candy bar back then was the Abba-Zaba bar. I wanted more than anything to make money so I could buy those.

So I started dumpster diving through the dumpsters behind the apartment complex where I lived, and I would fill trash bags up with cans. People who saw me do this probably thought I was some homeless scavenger. But I didn't care

60

what people thought of me because I was focused on getting money to buy candy.

I recruited my friend Brad to start doing the same thing with me. I convinced him that by working together we could earn enough money to buy as much candy as we wanted. When he joined in the effort, we started attacking the dumpsters every single day. They were like a goldmine to us, and we became obsessed with the whole process.

We'd fill up a bunch of bags worth of cans and plastic bottles, and we'd hook them over the handlebars of our Mongoose bikes and ride all the way across town to the recycling center. When we got there, we'd turn them in, and by the time they were all counted, we'd walk away with about eight bucks. We felt like we were rich because candy at that point cost 40 cents per bar.

I think this story is important because there's no doubt this was a dirty, gritty thing to do. But I was doing what I had to do to get what I wanted. When you're willing to do whatever you have to do to get what you want, people are going to look down on you. But you can have no shame. To this day, I would dive in a dumpster if I had to in order to reach a goal.

When you want something so bad in life that you would dive in any dumpster and swim through any sewer in order to get it, you can be sure that you're going to succeed. If you want something bad enough, there is nothing that can stand in your way.

When I was working as the fitness director at a health club and people were angry with me because I was moving equipment around and trying to train people in a better way, I didn't quit just because people were mad at me. I decided to do whatever I had to do in order to succeed.

What I had to do was take what I was doing and move it outside. I created something called Junkyard Gym. The only rules to Junkyard Gym were that you could not use any indoor equipment.

I returned to my roots to put this whole thing together. I went through dumpsters and pulled out milk cartons, crates and all kinds of random stuff to use as equipment. If someone was throwing away a dresser, I took it and used it as a step-up machine or a box jump.

What happened was Junkyard Gym got to be so popular that inside the 24,000 square foot health club, there were about 2 people left on any given day, and there were about 50 people outside training with me. This is when I realized that nobody cares about what equipment you have. Nobody cares about your pedigree. They only care about results. This is common sense, but we often forget this fact because it's not what we're taught.

Nobody cares about how much knowledge you have until they know how much you care and how committed you are to helping them do what they want to do. When I started

Junkyard Gym, I cared a lot about my clients, and I created an experience for them that brought people together.

I didn't know anything about business at the time, but I knew everything about creating teams. I knew how to create a strong culture. I knew there was power in that and power in creating a strong group of people focused on one common mission. That was one of the main things I learned playing sports.

As the popularity of my training at the gym increased, the goals the gym wanted me to hit kept getting bigger and bigger. What was happening was they saw that I was having success, and they wanted me to do more for them without working any more hours so they didn't have to pay me more.

I thought I was doing well. I was making a little over six figures, and I was still in my 20s. I felt rich because I'd been raised with a scarcity mindset. I'd been a part of a blue-collar family all of my life, and I liked the security I had with my job. I probably would have stayed and kept working for the same gym for a long time, but one of the fundamental things that was lacking was any kind of acknowledgement. I was not being acknowledged for what I was accomplishing whatsoever.

This is something I always say: bad companies don't take care of good people. Great companies, however, take care of great people. It's just like when you're on a team. A coach has to take care of the top producers on any team.

They've got to acknowledge when somebody does something good on the field or on the court.

The general manager didn't even know I had my own website. This was the guy working one level above me, and I worked with him every single day. But he never took an interest in what I was doing. He was disconnected from everything that was going on. He was not focused on the service I was providing or the mission I had undertaken to really help people. He was focused on the numbers. He didn't care anything about me, which was frustrating.

But I was still having a lot of success up until word got around that I was thinking about starting my own gym. Instead of deciding to back me in my training efforts, the health club I was working for decided to fire me. The regional director in our last meeting together told me, "Brian, I wish you the best of luck, but I have to be honest with you—I'm rooting against you, and I hope that you fail so you come back and work for us."

I didn't say a word in response to this, but I thought in my mind, "I'll never work for you again. If anything, you'll be working for me in the future." I went into football mode, the kill or be killed mentality my stepdad taught me. I knew I had to succeed, and I was willing to risk everything to give myself a shot at what I believed I deserved. I had to dive into the dumpster once again. I had to give up the security and in the end give more to other people to achieve what I wanted to achieve.

At the foundation of becoming more is giving more. When you give more and do more, you naturally become more. Many times, people want to work backwards. They want to be more from the start without having to do the work or give anything up. But to succeed, you have to give up the things that are blocking your way to success. This is the winning formula for anything you want to accomplish in your life. It's a scary, dirty process, but it's the only way I know that works.

Chapter Seven

Lesson

"Get Your Hands Dirty"

There is nothing more that I respect in a person than the willingness to get one's hands dirty at any cost to accomplish a mission. People with a "do whatever it takes" to accomplish something mentality are rare these days. Think of someone right now who is always willing to do things that many think are scary, gross, uncomfortable, or intimidating. We all know those one or two people who don't care what other people think of them and are constantly taking action.

If you look at anyone who has had major success in their life, chances are they've had many moments where they've had to sacrifice their ego and do what others would never do to accomplish what they have. One of the biggest factors that holds people back from going after what they want is their ego. For many people, the fear of what people will say about them is greater than the reward of achieving their goal. The reality is, no one cares. Literally, no one cares if you are willing to get dirty or make sacrifices to get what you want. Even if you are posting all over social media about it because you're proud of your grind, no one cares. The point is that you need to stay so focused on your missions that it doesn't matter if people praise you or hate on you.

Assuming you can elevate to great in any aspect of your life without getting dirty and being in the mud at times is lying to yourself. The dirtier you get and the deeper you go, the more you will grow.

Don't let the opinions of people who would never have the courage to step outside of their comfort zones affect your desire, decision, actions and will to become great. The real leaders will respect your hustle and drive to have a "whatever it takes" attitude. In order to succeed, you have to be willing to dive in, do the dirty work and give up your ego.

Game Changing Moves:

1. What is one thing you want so bad in your life right now that you would be willing to dive into any dumpster and get your hands dirty in order to get it?

2. How many of your day-to-day actions and risks you take to move you towards your goals are determined by how people will look at you?

3. Ask yourself, which is worse: Not accomplishing your goals and dreams? Or people laughing at you for trying?

(Please use the space below)

_____

_____

_____

_____

_____

_____

_____

_____

_____

_____

"At the foundation of becoming more is giving more."

#ElevatetoGreat

@CoachBrianNunez

Chapter 8

My Journey from the Bottom

Getting fired from the gym I was working at was not part of my plan. When it happened, I felt stuck. I didn't know anything about starting my own gym or even much about making money in general. I had a lot of clients who liked my approach to training them, but I didn't have a gym to work out of or any structure behind me anymore.

All I could do was take massive action. I didn't have time to mess around because my back was against the wall. This is why I believe the two best times in your life are when you're thriving, or when you're at rock bottom. When you're about to go bankrupt or die, it's like you're on your last life.

People often agree with me that it's great to be thriving, but they don't agree about rock bottom being a great place to be. But both of these places in life force you to make massive moves, though in different ways.

When you have momentum and success behind you, it makes you crave even more. It gives you the confidence to keep pushing the limit further. And when you're about to be dominated by life because of death, bankruptcy, a failed marriage or whatever problem you're facing, you are forced to do whatever it takes to succeed.

The worst place to be in life is right in the middle where things are not that bad, but they're also not that good. This is when you start to justify where you're at, and you just start treading water and getting nowhere. The best place to be is either at the bottom of the pool so you can push off the ground and shoot up like a rocket, or swimming with so much current behind you that you can't stop.

When I got fired, I was in the first position. I was at the bottom. I had no money coming in. I had a mortgage to pay, or I was going to lose my house. I had to figure everything out fast, or I wasn't just going to be diving into dumpsters—I was going to be living in one.

I had to be assertive and have meetings with a whole bunch of different people. I had to learn about conditional use permits, insurance, zoning—a whole list of stuff I had never even heard of before. It was overwhelming. I signed the lease on a warehouse, and I had to learn all the responsibilities that came with that.

I had no choice but to be ready and keep firing away. I had to go speak in front of the city council in my area about why I should be allowed to put a gym where I wanted to put one. Everything had to happen fast.

My girlfriend at the time (who is my wife now) was very supportive. She told me, "It's okay. If we have to lose the house, we have to lose the house." She was dedicated to being there beside me throughout the whole journey because she believed in my mission of helping other people. She believed that when you serve other people and give them what they need, you also are rewarded in your life.

She was my biggest support, but I also needed to expand my social circle to include more people who could help me. I had to surround myself with different people, and I had no room for negativity. I had no room for pessimism. I needed optimistic people who were smart and more educated than me to serve as my allies.

I had to go out and find these people because the truth is that you are the company you keep. Finding the right people to surround myself with was one of the things I did that helped me grow the most in business.

You can apply this idea to almost any area of your life. If you want to be more fit, go hang out with more fit people. People who are overweight hang out with people who are overweight. People who are fit hang out with people who are fit. People who make a lot of money hang out with people who make a lot of money, and people who are poor hang out with people who are poor.

When I started training at my warehouse with no equipment, money came in slowly at first. Some of my clients came with me from the start, others were used to training at a nice health club. They wanted to work with me, but they wanted to wait until I had my place set up and established.

I made enough money in the beginning just to pay my mortgage, put food on the table and pay my bills. I had no systems, organization, marketing or equipment, so I had to piece everything together as best as I could while I worked on those things. My clients were very accommodating during this whole process. They would come in and train in an empty warehouse with me.

I gave clients my energy, my authenticity and my principles. I saw that as long as I gave people results, and cared about their interests over mine, they could still get value from me. And this is where a lot of people get off track in so many areas of life. You have to continue to give everyone in your life the same level of care regardless of circumstances. This principle applies to relationships and marriage as well as business and coaching.

You have to treat your significant other with the same level of care as you did when you first started dating. You have to give your children your time, patience and love every day. If you're a business owner, you have to treat your employees well and not take them for granted. It's easy to slip into complacency, but if you do, you're giving up the only thing that matters. When you show other people that you care about what you do, and you care about helping them, you're on the path to true success.

Chapter Eight

Lesson

"Take Massive Action"

No matter what stage you are at in your life right now, there will come a time when you are extremely tested and challenged. It may be by a death, loss of a job, relationship problems, health problems, or any unfortunate, unexpected event in your life. The important thing to remember is to own your journey and that your "rock bottom" moment is unique to you. There is no need to compare your situation with anyone else's, what they did, or how they handled it. The focus needs to be on how you're going to handle adversity when it strikes.

We learn a lot about ourselves when we are backed into a corner and faced with a fight or flight moment. Do you face the issue head on? Do you accept and acknowledge the problem at hand, with no judgment, and plan your next move? Or do you make excuses, complain, and wonder why this happened to you? In every situation, you have two choices, and when you pick the first option, to accept and acknowledge the problem at hand, you will be more clear-headed and able to start taking massive action.

Massive action will always be the solution for change. When you are committed to solving a problem at any cost, willing to get your hands dirty, willing to reach out for help, and willing to do whatever it takes to get something done, it is almost impossible not to succeed.

Life is going to throw major curve balls at your game plan. Be grateful for those curveballs because challenges will make you grow. When dealing with any type of adversity, focus your energy on your strengths and get back to what you do best. Maybe you are a great coach or teacher who provides superior service to those you help, or maybe you are an athlete who has a strong work ethic, maniacal focus and dedication. It doesn't matter what you're best at, when you choose to take massive action in adversity, you always come out stronger than before.

Life is like working out and building your muscles; the more resistance you face and the more challenges you go through, the more you grow. The key to elevating from any "bottom level" in your life is to go all in and take massive action!

Game Changing Moves:

1. Where are you treading water in your life right now? Where is it in your life that things aren't that bad, but aren't that great?

2. Make a decision to ELEVATE, and take massive action to create positive momentum in your life.

3. What is one thing you can do to propel yourself towards elevation?

(Please use the space below)

_____

_____

_____

_____

_____

_____

_____

_____

_____

_____

_____

"The worst place to be in life is right in the middle where things are not that bad, but they're also not that good."

#ElevatetoGreat
@CoachBrianNunez

Chapter 9

The Importance of Developing Your Core Values

When I first opened up my gym, I started with about 30 clients. This was in 2011, and what I was doing with group training was a brand-new business model. This was before CrossFit and other small, boutique gyms were on every corner.

I was 27 years old, and I was trying to figure out how to succeed with the passion, purpose and care I talked about in the last chapter. I was a workhorse trying to help people as best as I could. I didn't know all the ins and outs of running a business, but I was fortunate to have a strong business partner.

He was not very much into fitness at the time, but he understood how things should be set up. He was very influential and helpful in the first two years of the business, but he let me run it for the most part. I'm grateful for this because it allowed me to see my areas of weakness and what I needed to improve upon as a leader and entrepreneur. If I hadn't had the chance to earn my battle scars in the thick of the fight, I would have never learned the real landscape and sport of business.

When it comes to learning how to take care of my employees, running good meetings and keeping my company strong, I look back at the leader I was in the early days of my business, and who I am now compared to who I was then is like night and day.

One of the biggest things I learned was that leadership is about being able to empathize with the people you're leading. When you can relate and empathize with somebody, that makes all the difference in the world. I had to learn this to better help my team and also to better serve my clients.

Some clients would say things to me like, "Dude, Brian, you're fit. You're an athlete, and you have been your entire life. You don't understand our struggle." And they were right. I didn't understand what it was like to be overweight. I didn't understand what it was like not to even be able to do a push up. I had to get into my clients' world to understand what it was like to do something I was not good at and even scared of doing, something I had no experience with.

What I decided to do to have this experience was I decided to run a marathon with my clients. This was way out of my comfort zone because I'm a sprinter. If you take a sprinter and make them run a marathon, you're putting them into a whole new ballgame.

When I ran the Boston Marathon in 2012, it was the most humbling physical experience of my life. I remember being at mile 21, and I had just gotten past what they call Heartbreak Hill, one of the most difficult parts of the race. I had five miles left to run, and I felt like somebody had taken a shotgun to my legs.

It felt like my body was shutting down. I kept moving, but I was moving at such a slow pace that little old ladies were running past me, patting me on the back and saying, "It's okay, honey. You're doing good." I didn't feel like I was doing good at all. I didn't believe I was going to be able to make it across the finish line, but I crossed it. I didn't enjoy it at all, but I made it to my goal.

I believe that I can't coach someone through something unless I've gone through their struggles and felt their pain myself. I couldn't coach people on how to live a fit, focused and free life if I had never gone through depression, identity crisis and emotional disconnection. I wouldn't be able to teach people how to create a successful business if I had never done it, or show people how to become physically fit if I myself wasn't fit.

For me, my standards and principles are that I have to practice what I preach. And the root of that is knowing my values, who I am, and what I am best positioned to help other people accomplish in their own lives.

Most people don't know their own values. You may know what you want in life, but you also have to understand what you value most. Throughout my life, there have been a lot of things that I wanted, but I didn't actually value them.

I wanted awards, popularity, and shiny objects, but in my heart those weren't even things I truly valued on a deeper level. I didn't care about them. I didn't even enjoy the attention when I got it, and I didn't enjoy who I was becoming when I chased after the illusions instead of living a life true to myself.

The first step to living a free life is to ask yourself what really matters to you. Does a Lamborghini matter to you? Maybe, maybe not. Does owning a private jet matter to you? Maybe, maybe not.

There's no right or wrong answer to these types of questions, but they deserve consideration, or you may find yourself working blindly towards someone else's idea of success. Your core values are what center you and give you fulfillment. When you start living and following your values, that's when you begin to understand your worth.

My number one core value is to be authentic and to live an authentic life. I want to live me and who I'm designed to be, because I understand the pain that comes from not doing that. I've seen the problems living with no connection to yourself can cause. It can be devastating.

Number two is to play with passion. No matter what I'm doing, I want to do it with effort and a positive attitude. If I'm sweeping the floor, or if I'm connecting with somebody, I want to give them all of my energy, passion and enthusiasm. I don't want to do anything half-heartedly. To me, that's a huge waste of time.

Number three is to practice what I preach. I have absolutely no tolerance for hypocrites in life. I hate them. I hate people who talk the talk and don't walk the walk. I never, ever want to be that person. For me to be able to relate with people, I have to be a person of honesty and integrity. That means I never want to say one thing and do another.

Number four is to provide consistent communication. This plays a role both when it comes to communicating with myself, and also communicating with other people. If you don't consistently communicate with yourself, and you don't audit yourself, you will have a bad relationship with yourself. The same goes for your relationships with other people. If there's not constant communication, feedback and connection being made, you will not have a good relationship with someone else.

My last core value is to protect my tribe at all costs. This means to take care of my family and to take care of the people who I work with and train with every single day. I want to make sure I leave this earth on great terms with every single person I care about. I want them to know my intention is to help them and be there for them.

I have lived in opposition to every single one of my core values at some point in my life. But the experience of not living a life aligned with what I believe is right is what has brought me to the point of understanding the importance of continually dedicating myself to living by my core values.

You need to write down as many core values as you feel you want to live by. For some people, that may be three. For some it may be 20. The simplest way to do this is to first write down all of the things you can say with 100% conviction you do not want in your life. Then you can write down the values you need to have to avoid those things.

Your values are your signposts. Design them to guide you away from what you don't want in your life and towards what you do want. When you create your list of core values, some of them may be obvious. Some of them may take a long time to develop, and that's okay. The important thing is that you continually dedicate yourself to a life guided by them, even when you experience momentary failure.

Chapter Nine

Lesson

"Knowing What Matters Most"

The root of success is knowing what matters most to you and living out your values every day. Although we live in a society where success is defined as having a certain job title, money, a nice house, fancy cars, and many other materialistic things, real success starts with living your truth. Knowing who you are and what is important to you is the first step to winning the game of life.

There are two types of people who react very differently when they walk into a crowded room. One type feels that no matter how many people are there, they are lost and alone. They seek to be around other people for security and comfort, and yet, this never truly satisfies their desire to feel seen and validated. The other type of person feels content in a crowded place. They feel no need to "fit in" and are calm and confident. They enjoy their own company and presence, alone or in a crowded room.

For many years, I struggled with being the first person. No matter how exciting or crowded a party or event was, I still felt alone. I constantly needed to be with other people for validation and security. It wasn't until I took the time to write down not only what was most important to me, but also what I was no longer willing to tolerate in my life that my life changed. For most people, writing down their core values is an extremely hard thing to do; it can actually be pretty scary for some. The best way to come up with them is to think about what you don't want in your life and create values that will steer you in the opposite direction.

Knowing what you value most in life is the key to understanding yourself, your worth, and how you are uniquely positioned to serve others. Your core values are the principles that you choose to live by. You can have as many of them as you want, but they must be standards you are willing to uphold no matter what. Creating your core values is the foundation to elevating to greatness in any and every aspect of your life!

Game Changing Moves:

1. Make a list of all the things you know for sure you do not want in your life. (Negativity, passivity, gossip, lying, etc.)

2. Make a list of the pain and cost of allowing these negative things to be in your life.

3. Make your values list. Write down what you value most in life and how you want to live your life.

(Please use the space below)

_____

_____

_____

_____

_____

_____

_____

_____

_____

_____

_____

"When you start living and following your values, that's when you begin to understand your worth."

#ElevatetoGreat

@CoachBrianNunez

Chapter 10

The Peanut Butter and Jelly Vision

Having a vision for your life is all about imagining the possibilities. Your vision guides you towards the life you want to live. To create your vision, you have to first start off with a dream. Your dream is the seed of what is to come. Most people don't have trouble with this first step.

A lot of people find it easy to live in dreamland. When you get bored in class or at work, you might start thinking about all the things you would rather be doing with your life. This isn't necessarily a bad thing, but it's not going to produce any results for you unless you move on to step two.

Step two is to visualize the dream in your actual life. This means to make the dream a reality in your mind to where you can see it, smell it, taste it and feel it. You make it real in your mind before it's in front of you in reality. Then you ask yourself, "Do I believe it's possible? Do I believe I'm worth it? Do I believe I can achieve it?" Now, once you get over the belief hump, step three is to go after it. You've got to become maniacally focused and cut the brakes. You've got to go for it 100%. There's no more second-guessing or backing down allowed at this point.

One of the visions I have for my life is to help 10 million people all over the world become more fit in all aspects of their lives—physically, mentally, and emotionally. I want to help them live a focused and free life through my programs, products and coaching. I can see this vision very clearly, and I believe in it 100%.

The purpose behind why I want to do this is because I believe in paying it forward. I believe in making an impact in other people's lives. There are many reasons why I want to do this, but there's one particular story I want to share with you about how I came to want to help as many people on the face of this earth as possible.

When I was a kid, my parents would always pack me the same thing for lunch. They'd pack me a peanut butter and jelly sandwich, a Capri Sun, and sometimes a bag of chips on a good day.

My buddies at school always had all these extra things like Fruit Roll Ups, Gushers, and other fancy little snacks. I wanted that kind of stuff in my lunch so bad, and I was always jealous of what they had. I remember I was always ungrateful that all I had was a peanut butter and jelly sandwich.

If I could go back and change my attitude, I would. I was lucky to have parents that would make me a lunch every single day, but I didn't see it that way at the time.

As the years passed, I headed off to college, and I started making myself peanut butter and jelly sandwiches for lunch. I was on my own for the first time, and I didn't really know how to cook, so it just seemed right. It was ingrained in my head that eating a peanut butter and jelly sandwich for lunch was just what I did.

I went to college at San Jose State, and I lived downtown near a park called Saint James Park. For lunch, I'd make myself a sandwich, and then I'd go walk through the park every single day. As I walked through the park, I saw a lot of homeless people and people who were having a tough go in life. I remember one day as I was walking, a guy came up to me and asked me, "Hey, man, can I have some money?"

I was a broke college student. I didn't have any money at the time, so I told him, "Sorry, I have no money. The only thing I have on me is this peanut butter and jelly sandwich."

To which the guy responded, "Oh my gosh, man, I would love that. PB&J reminds me of my childhood." I'll never forget what the guy said next. He said, "I really appreciate this, man. It's more than just a sandwich. You made me feel at home."

This stuck with me because I felt the exact same way, but I'd never been able to articulate it. A peanut butter and jelly sandwich was comfort for me because for so many years my parents had put so much love into making sure I had a lunch every day. As a kid, I didn't understand that. But when this guy said that the sandwich made him feel at home, something just clicked inside me.

After this experience, I was inspired to help more people that I saw struggling. I still didn't have much to give, but I started to make extra sandwiches to take with me on my walk through the park. I wanted to give more people in tough situations a sense of being cared for and thought about.

This is why when I started my company, I wanted to continue to help other people in need. I want all the athletes who work with me to know the importance of paying it forward and helping others. To me, doing this is an important part of living a healthy life. Your focus can't just be on you. You've got to do something to give back.

There are different ways to do this. One way is to donate money to causes that are important to you. But the other even more important way to do this is by doing something directly to help other people in your community. This is why I started something called Peanut Butter and Jelly Day.

What we do is once a month, the whole community rallies around our mission to give back, and we go to different local homeless shelters in the area and hand out peanut butter and jelly sandwiches. It's very rewarding because what we're doing is not just handing out food. We're handing out love, comfort and a sense of home.

Last year, we had a giving goal of 10,000 sandwiches. We wanted to impact the lives of 10,000 people, and we surpassed that. We gave out 11,000. None of this would be possible if it was just me trying to do this on my own. Back when I was a college student, I wanted to help in a big way, but I didn't have the means to do it. But I kept it in my mind that I would one day be able to, and I'm grateful for all the people who have now come along side me to help make this vision a reality.

When people are aligned with the same vision of giving back and paying it forward, big things happen. This is why having a vision for the life you want to live is important. The life you choose to live will impact others, and when you join forces and share a vision for a better world with those around you, you will send ripples of positivity, love and care throughout your community and beyond.

Chapter Ten

Lesson

"Dream Big with a Clear Vision"

The first step to creating a vision for your life is to dream big! You weren't meant for an average or normal life; you were meant for greatness. Go back to the child inside of you, who used to dream that anything was possible when you were younger. Before people, media, and outside sources told you to be "realistic" and "practical." The path to elevating to greatness is dreaming so big that it inspires you to make your dreams a reality.

The second step is to visualize your dreams coming true in your actual life and make them as real as possible in your mind. You must believe 100% that they are actually possible. This is the **Power of Visualization**. It has to be so clear in your mind and heart that you feel as if you have already accomplished it. You must feed your vision daily with written goals and images to help enhance your inspiration to make it become a reality.

The third step is to become obsessed with making your dream a reality and take massive action towards what you want to see happen. Your vision for your life is ultimately not just about *you*, because paying it forward and giving back are a major part of living a healthy life. The greatest impact you can make on the world occurs when you share your vision with others and everyone works together to see it become a reality. There is no such thing as a person who is "self-made." Every person that you meet along your journey will have an impact on you and the legacy you leave.

In order to make your vision come to life, you must see it, believe it, and then be it…every day!

Game Changing Moves:

1. If you could accomplish anything you wanted in life, what would it be? Write it down.
2. How would it make you feel to live the life you've always dreamed of?
3. What impact would you want to make in other people's lives?

(Please use the space below)

_____

_____

_____

_____

_____

_____

_____

_____

_____

_____

_____

"Your focus can't just be on you. You've got to do something to give back."

#ElevatetoGreat
@CoachBrianNunez

Chapter 11

The Four C's to Freedom

Living a free life is an inside job. What I mean is that becoming free is only possible if you focus and make changes on the inside. There are four steps to this process. I call them the four C's.

The first C is *Clarity*. This involves knowing your vision, your mission and what actions you must take to accomplish your mission. Most people believe that once they know what they want to accomplish and how to accomplish it, it's going to be smooth sailing from there. But that's not how it works because what happens is as you try to progress forward, you are given a whole different set of problems to deal with. Problems you didn't even know were problems.

This is where clarity becomes really important. You have to be able to paint the picture and see exactly where you're going and what your destination is. This is the only way to get the monkey off your back. That monkey is uncertainty.

Uncertainty is the giant gorilla that holds people back because they aren't clear on what they want. They don't know their roots. They don't know enough about themselves in order to see what's beyond the uncertainty.

Now, once you have clarity, and you can see exactly what you're going after, the next C is **Conviction**. Conviction means not swaying from the goal you've chosen for yourself. There's no "on the fence" about what you're doing.

I'm naturally a hardcore people pleaser. I want to make everybody happy. It used to be that when somebody asked me to do something, I would automatically say yes. I said yes because I didn't want to disappoint anyone. I went to all the barbecues, parties, and events that people asked me to go to, but the problem was I didn't actually want to do all of these things.

My wife noticed this was an issue for me first, and she said to me, "Brian, the problem is you don't know how to say no. But you have to realize that when you say no, your yes becomes more powerful." I was saying yes to everything and wearing myself thin. I wasn't putting much energy into anything I was doing because I was exhausting myself.

When I started saying no, people realized that when I said yes it meant I was all in. Now when I say yes, people know I'm going to give 110%, not 30%. This is where conviction comes in. You can only know when to say no when you know what you want in life.

Your values help you determine this. When you know your vision and mission, it becomes super easy for you to say no to the things that do not align with it. I had to learn this through experience. I lived the majority of my life as an opportunist. Now I live my life as a strategist. An opportunist says yes to every opportunity. They don't consider whether something is in line with their vision or not.

Now, for someone who is just starting out in life, it's not necessarily a bad thing to be an opportunist. If you don't know for sure what you want because you haven't had any experience doing anything, then experience is a valuable way to gain clarity. But your goal with this should be to get to the point of conviction so it is easy for you to know where to draw the line.

The third C stands for **Courage**. I don't believe that anybody is born with courage. Courage requires action. It requires you to overcome fear, and it requires you to do things you don't want to do. When you are challenged, being courageous is about moving through those challenges and doing what you have to do to succeed.

One of the biggest ways to be courageous is to allow yourself to be held accountable for your actions. When you allow a mentor or coach to hold you to a higher standard, you're being courageous. It takes a lot of courage to allow a coach to peer into your life and point out your flaws and what you need to work on.

Some of the coaches I have right now scare the shit out of me. I have to exercise courage just to have them be a part of my life because I know they're not going to let me get away with anything. They have one job, and that is to make me better and hold me accountable.

The last C is **Consistency**. What happens for the majority of people is they have all of the other three C's down for short periods of time. They have clarity, conviction and courage for a while, but then they get off track. People often tell me how they used to be in great shape, but then one day they stopped eating right, exercising and taking care of themselves.

This is why consistency is what ties everything together. Without it, you can't achieve freedom in your life. Consistency is king—not intensity. Consistency trumps intensity any day of the week. The people who keep chipping away at their masterpiece and shaping it while the whole world is trying to distract them are the ones who have long-term success in whatever they're trying to achieve.

This is why it's so important to surround yourself with the kinds of people who work this way. Get away from the people who will try to distract you from your goals. Be mission-driven, focus-driven and understand why you're doing what you're doing.

There will be times when you will question why you're working so hard, and everyone has those thoughts. But when you refocus on your values and the war you're trying to win, then you get yourself back into the game. You keep going. You might have slowed down, but when you jump back in, you increase your speed.

That's why every single one of the four C's is important. You want to crush it not once, not twice, but over and over for the rest of your life. Don't ever give up.

Chapter Eleven

Lesson

"Freedom Requires Clarity, Conviction, Courage and Consistency"

Freedom begins with the changes that you make on the inside. There are four steps to this process of change. The first C is Clarity. You have to know exactly what you want so when you're challenged, you can still see the end goal that you're working towards. Once you have created your values and the vision for your life, your purpose will become more clear. As perfectly stated by Malcolm X, "If you don't stand for something, you will fall for anything." Knowing who you are, what you value, and what mission you are on helps drive and bring clarity to your purpose.

The second C is Conviction. You have to have strong conviction when operating from the set of core values that you believe in. If something is not aligned with your values, don't say yes to it. Most people have a hard time saying NO to people or opportunities. But when you have conviction in your mission and KNOW exactly what you want, you will never have a hard time saying no to things that don't align with your strategy.

The third C is Courage. Courage requires you to face your fears and move through them head on. You have to do what scares you in order to keep growing. Have the courage to be committed to greatness at all costs. There will be times when things don't go according to plan, but it will be your courage to stay committed, even when faced with obstacle after obstacle, that will get you through and bring you one step closer to what you want.

The fourth C is Consistency. You will not achieve freedom in your life unless you keep chipping away at it. Consistency trumps intensity. Don't ever give up. When you fail, get back up and try even harder. When you succeed, never settle or be satisfied, and always have the mindset that your best is yet to come. Your consistency will be the deciding factor of whether or not you achieve any goal in your life.

Game Changing Moves:

1. Which of the four C's do you need to spend more focus and energy on in your life?
2. Write down one goal you have for your life.
3. Say it out loud as if you have already accomplished it.
4. Be courageous enough to share it with someone who will hold you accountable.
5. Do steps 2-4 everyday. You get what you repeatedly do!

(Please use the space below)

_____

_____

_____

_____

_____

_____

_____

_____

_____

_____

"Living free is an inside job."

#ElevatetoGreat

@CoachBrianNunez

Chapter 12

Build Your Super Hero Squad

A super hero squad is different than your social circle. Your social circle might be your friends, family and the people you're around from day to day. Your super hero squad is who you have assembled around you to get you to the next level. To assemble it, you have to have clarity, conviction, courage and consistency operating in your life. You have to know exactly what you value. You have to know your strengths. What do you bring to the team?

When you know your strengths, then you're ready to build your superhero squad. But you shouldn't build your super hero squad around your strengths. You should build your superhero squad around your weaknesses. When you have others filling in your weaknesses with their strengths, then you can accomplish much more in much less time.

When it comes to my squad, I don't need another Brian. I don't need somebody to come in and light a fire and energize my team because that's what I do. That's my special ability. But I do I need somebody who can look at the details, stay organized and keep everything together because that's a weakness of mine.

When you're going through the process of building your team, you have to be humble enough to know what you're not good at. You have to be able to recognize your weaknesses.

Focusing on your strengths is important because that builds confidence, but that's just part of the picture. If you don't acknowledge your weaknesses, you won't be able to identify who you need on your squad to counteract those weaknesses.

You don't want to just focus on your weaknesses, but they need to be identified. Don't stay with them too long because where your focus goes, that's where energy flows. Focusing on your weaknesses constantly will make you weaker. But acknowledging them and counteracting them with someone else's strengths makes good things happen.

When it comes to any organization I'm working with, I don't try to bring people on board that all have the exact same strengths. Not only is that very difficult to do, it also weakens the team. Diversity on a team is what leads to longer-lasting success. And the leader of every team must operate with transparency, trust and understanding of exactly what each member is best at.

Once your squad is set, you've got all the weapons you will need to win the battle. You've got all the resources and help you need, so the next thing you have to do is bet on yourself.

When you've identified your strengths and know what you bring to the table, then you have to believe in your heart that you will produce results for your team. It doesn't matter if you've done what you're trying to do before or not. All that matters is that you believe strongly that you can succeed in the area that other people are counting on you in. Let me give you a little story to illustrate what I mean.

When I was younger, I wasn't surrounded by people who had a lot of money. I didn't see people going on vacations, driving luxury cars or flying jets. To me, all of that was fantasy. That was all stuff I only saw in movies.

But when I moved into Silicon Valley, suddenly life looked like a whole different ball game. A lot of people in this area have a lot of wealth. And I remember starting to train clients who were CEOs and CFOs and people with titles I didn't even understand the meaning of.

It was crazy to me when these clients started asking me to go with them on trips, fly in their jets, and do stuff that felt extravagant. I didn't understand why they wanted me to do all this stuff with them, because hanging out with them didn't feel like my scene. It was a little uncomfortable.

But one of my clients told me something that changed everything. He told me, "Brian, you have a gift. People want to be around you because you're rich in energy and positivity.

You're rich in health, and while you may feel uncomfortable surrounded by money and luxury, you're rich in other ways. That's why I want you in my life—for the value that you bring to it."

It was at this point that I understood the word rich was about more than money. My value to people didn't have to do with the money I had in my pocket. They didn't want me around for my bank account. They wanted me around because I was able to provide something that they needed in their lives.

You must also recognize what your strengths are and how they can be valuable to others. You have valuable traits and skills that you can bring to the table with your squad. So put all your chips on the table, and bet on your ability to be strong in areas where others are weak. When you do this, your team will respond. Your energy will be contagious, and you will end up with a super hero squad capable of achieving its mission.

Chapter Twelve

Lesson

"Assemble Your Allies"

One of the biggest contributors to your success will be the allies that you have in your life. This group of A+ players will not only support you in your journey, but also will hold you accountable to raising your standards to greatness. Align yourself with people who do not make excuses and are not looking for average, people who are hand-picked and assembled by you for one reason: to help you elevate to great in your life.

Your super hero squad are the different people you've assembled around you to help you get to the next level. In order to assemble who you need on your squad, you must first recognize and identify your weaknesses. This is because you need to choose people to join your squad whose strengths are your weaknesses. You don't want to find people who all have the same strengths. Diversity on a team is what leads to lasting success. When you understand the value that you bring to the table, then go all in on bringing your strengths to the team in order to achieve its mission. When you fully commit as a leader, your squad will follow suit.

You are the company you keep. If you are the smartest person in the room, you are in the wrong room. You will know you are in the right place in life when your superhero squad makes you feel slightly uncomfortable, because you know that they will always put their best foot forward and expect you to do the same. Your life will dramatically change when you start to surround yourself with people who want to win as badly as you do.

Game Changing Moves:

1. Make a list of all of your strengths. What are all of the things that you naturally do well?
2. Make a list of your weaknesses. What are all of the things that you do not do well?
3. Make a list of the people you know (not just personally) whose strengths are your weaknesses.
4. Assemble your super hero squad!

(Please use the space below)

_____

_____

_____

_____

_____

_____

_____

_____

_____

_____

"You have to be humble enough to know what you're not good at, and you have to be able to recognize your weaknesses."

#ElevatetoGreat
@CoachBrianNunez

Chapter 13

Burn the Boats

When I first started my business, I knew nothing about the ins and outs of running a successful gym. But I bet on my commitment, authenticity and desire to help other people out in a genuine, positive way. I knew I could win in the game of business even though in the beginning, every day I would walk into an empty warehouse.

I didn't even have equipment for the first few months. There was no music playing, but I stood there, and I could hear the music. I could see the high fives, the people working hard towards their goals.

Before anybody even knew who I was and what I was doing, I believed I would succeed. I didn't even have a name for my business, and nothing was established yet, but I bet on myself because I knew that the only way I was going to lose was if I died. I was willing to fail 50 times in order to get it right one time.

Seven years later, and we're now the top training facility in the Bay Area which is one of the hardest markets to succeed in because it's one of the healthiest city in America.

We have tons of competition, but the difference is we hold nothing back. We give people our all every single day, and that's what people are looking for.

What holds most people back is insecurity. Insecurity causes people to say things like, "Well, if this doesn't work out, then at least I have this other opportunity." But this is the worst way to look at things because it means you're living on the fence. You're treading water. If you don't give all of yourself to something, then the return you're going to get in the end is going to be microscopic. It's going to end up being the equivalent of what you've invested.

This is why I live with a burn the boats mentality. Having a burn the boats mentality means you're not even going to entertain the possibility of failure or taking the easy way out. You can't keep one foot in the past when you're trying to accomplish something new. You have to commit fully to the vision, and you can't look back and second-guess yourself.

There are a few key concepts I think are incredibly important for anyone building a business. The first is that you can't believe the haters, and the second is that you can't believe the hype. To burn the boats, you can't believe the people who doubt you, and you can't believe that it's ever okay to stop continuously improving.

I went skydiving a few years back, and when I jumped out of the plane, I had no way of knowing what was going to happen. It was a scary, but exhilarating experience. The way I viewed it, I was either going to fail and die, or I was going to survive and be able to tell the incredible story of how I jumped out of a plane. There was no in-between or gray area about what the result was going to be. Those were the two options.

Now, the reality is that most things you will attempt in life do not have life or death consequences. When you take the risk and leave a bad relationship, that's not a life or death thing. Neither is taking the risk to start a business. The worst that can happen is you lose the business.

When you burn the boats, you assume 100% responsibility for everything in your life. If you choose to start a business, how then can it fail? If you assume responsibility for everything, the only way your business can fail is if you lack the dedication and commitment required to find a way to make it succeed.

If you are your only problem, then you are your only solution. This is the mentality that I have. If things are going wrong, it's because of me. I have either not committed enough, not invested enough or I'm playing it safe. And I have to become the solution in all of these scenarios.

If something goes wrong in my company, maybe 10 people did something wrong, but I take responsibility for not training them properly. If something isn't going right in my marriage, I take responsibility—maybe I didn't make it my obsession to make sure my wife and I spent quality time together.

If something goes wrong between my daughter and I, I look at what I did to contribute to the issue. Did I give her my full attention when we were together? When I go home every night, I put my phone away when I have dinner with my daughter. I get rid of that distraction, that boat that takes me somewhere else, and I focus my attention fully on her.

Burning the boats in your life is all about creating balance. This doesn't mean that you do everything at the same time in small doses. That's not real balance. The kind of balance I'm talking about means going all in on one thing in your life when you're doing that one thing. And when you're done with that, you focus 100% on the next thing

When I'm having a conversation with my wife, I'm 100% engaged in that conversation. When I'm talking to my daughter, I'm 100% engaged in being the best dad I can possibly be. When I'm working on social media for my business, I'm obsessed with giving that my whole attention.

Achieving balance is not about giving 10% here, 15% there and 75% over there. Balance comes from doing one thing 100% when you're doing that one thing, and doing it 0% when you're focused on something else. Your attention is your greatest asset. Don't waste it by spreading it thin.

Chapter Thirteen

Lesson

"Go all in...100/1"

If you don't give all of yourself to something, then the return you're going to get from it is going to be microscopic. You must give 100% of your attention and effort to the one thing you choose to do, hence 100/1. Being balanced is not about doing ten things at once. Being balanced is about doing only one thing at a time, and then shifting your focus to the next thing when the time comes for you to move on.

Often times people use the term "balance" when they actually mean "presence." It's impossible to focus your energy on two things at the same time while being fully present. The idea that multi-tasking is a good thing is one of the biggest lies we have ever been told. When people are more present in the current moment that they're in, not getting distracted by their phones or other things going on around them, but rather fully engaging and giving their undivided attention to someone or something, that is when they achieve balance. This is necessary to do in order to go all in on your goals and *burn the boats*.

When you burn the boats, you are going all in on whatever you're trying to accomplish. You're accepting full

119

responsibility for all of your results or failures. There is no turning back. You have fully committed and need to have the awareness, engagement, and commitment to stay focused and achieve your goals. Success is the only option. Because, at the end of the day, you are your only problem, and you are your only solution. When you take on this belief, the actions you must take in any situation become obvious. You are the only one who can decide if you will succeed or if you will fail. Choose wisely.

Game Changing Moves:

1. What is one area of your life that you need to fully commit to and burn the boats?

2. Write down three things you can do to hold yourself more accountable to being more focused on your missions.

(Please use the space below)

_____

_____

_____

_____

_____

_____

_____

_____

_____

_____

"You are your only problem, and you are your only solution."

#ElevatetoGreat

@CoachBrianNunez

Chapter 14

The Three Pillars of Health

Sometimes when I have a room full of clients, I ask them, "Who here in this room is rich?" Most of the time, nobody raises their hand. Then I tell them, "No one is raising their hand because you all have been brainwashed to believe that being rich has to do with money, but being rich in health is way more important."

We all need to reprogram our minds because being rich in physical health is the most important thing we could ever focus on, and it's actually very simple. I get hundreds of messages and emails every single day from people asking me if I can help them get into better shape because people are confused. They don't know what's good advice because the world has overcomplicated the whole process of getting healthy and staying healthy.

There are thousands of different diets and workouts all claiming to be the best. It's not that these don't work, but when you focus on complicated diets and workout routines, you make health way more complicated than it needs to be.

Everything you need to know to become rich in health can be broken down into three major things. The first and most important part of your physical health is your mindset. Your software controls your hardware. Your hardware is a byproduct of the wiring of your software. If you want to have strong software, aka a strong mindset, there are two things you need to do.

Number one, you need to sleep for at least seven hours a night minimum. Sleep is the most underrated thing when it comes to weight loss, stress levels and productivity. This isn't talked about much. In fact, sleep is often the first thing people cut out when they decide they're going to work harder and try to achieve more in their lives.

If you believe you don't need sleep, then you're not taking care of yourself. You might be able to survive on hardly any sleep for 10 years, but eventually you're going to burn yourself into the ground.

The second part of the mindset portion is you need to write down your goals daily. One of my spiritual mentors taught me that attention is our greatest asset like I mentioned in the last chapter. In order to make a change in life, the only thing that's needed is heightening of your attention.

Writing down your goals focuses your attention on one area, and this makes everything you do flow out of that. When your attention is heightened to see what you really want, it becomes easier for you to make the right choices.

If I were to ask you to write down your weight loss goals, and you said you wanted to lose 5% body fat, and then we went out to lunch, and you had the option to choose between a plate of broccoli and chicken and a plate full of pizza, which one would you choose? The answer is obvious. You would choose the chicken and broccoli because your attention would still be focused on your weight loss goal.

This ties right into the second most important part of your physical health, and that is your meals—what you eat. The truth is that you already know what is healthy for you to eat and what is not healthy for you to eat. The problem is that it's so easy to lose focus and attention. 16 hours of each day you are awake and in a ready state. For those 16 hours, you have to make decisions. The other eight hours you are asleep and recharging.

If you're in a bad state of mind during the 16 hours you have to make decisions, your decisions are going to be bad. Your nutrition is directly related to your attention and the decisions you make because of it. Eating well doesn't require Atkins, intermittent fasting, Paleo or any other crazy diet. I've never followed a meal plan in my entire life because eating is just a byproduct of behavior.

When you know that behavior controls your eating, and your behavior is controlled by what you focus on, you get to the root of the problem. This is why my "meal plan" has always been simple. My meal plan is called the D.E.S. meal plan. D.E.S. stands for Don't. Eat. Shit.

All you have to do to follow this meal plan is ask yourself one question before every meal you eat: Is this meal going to help me achieve my goal, or is it going to hurt me? When you make yourself answer this question, then you have the power of responsibility. You have taken responsibility for your goal. If you don't like your results, and yet you keep making the decision to eat food you know is unhealthy over and over, then you know what needs to change.

If you drink half of your body weight in water every single day, and eat 10 to 12 servings of vegetables a day, your health is guaranteed to improve. This is the simplest plan you could ever follow, and it works.

The last major component of physical health is movement. When it comes to movement and exercise, whatever you will do consistently will produce results. Consistency trumps intensity. Going hard in the gym for two weeks like you're Michael Jordan isn't going to change a thing.

All you have to do is spend 30 minutes a day exercising. Do whatever exercise you enjoy doing the most and will consistently do. For example, if someone told me to get in shape by cycling, I wouldn't be able to do it because I don't like cycling. But I could get in shape by playing basketball or lifting weights because those are things I do enjoy.

What I've discussed in this chapter are the three pillars of becoming rich in health. To recap, they are mindset, meals and movement. These are the only three things that matter. Don't overcomplicate things. Keep things simple, and most of all stay consistent in your efforts.

Chapter Fourteen

Lesson

"Keep it Simple and Sustainable"

Many people are confused when it comes to knowing what they need to do to get healthy. This is because the world has overcomplicated things. There are so many diets and exercises out there that claim to be the best, but the truth is that getting healthy does not have to be a complicated process. There are three pillars to health. The first is your mindset. Your mindset determines what choices you make, and your choices are what impact your health. You must prioritize sleep to maintain a healthy mindset, but you must also write down your goals daily so they are at the top of your mind. If you want to maximize your focus each day, write your goals down twice a day, once in the morning and once at night. This will help you create a productive day and avoid doing "busy" work. When you write your big goals down two times a day, you aren't allowing yourself to get sidetracked by things that are insignificant. Every action we take is derived from our focus, or lack thereof. Set yourself up to win by constantly setting your compass for success.

The second pillar is your meals. My meal plan is simple. D.E.S.—Don't. Eat. Shit. This may seem blunt, but there is nothing more honest than this. The reality is we know what is healthy and what is unhealthy. The problem most people face is that their nutrition is tied to their behavior and their behavior is tied to their focus. Writing down your goals twice a day gets to the root of the problem and helps align your focus and shift your behavior to a positive, healthy state. Ask yourself one question before every meal, "Will this help me or hurt me in achieving my goals?" Take ownership of how you fuel your body.

The last pillar is your movement. There are no magic exercises that help transform your body. The only exercises that have a profound effect on your body are the exercises that you enjoy doing and will do *consistently*. Consistency trumps intensity. Get on a consistent training plan that combines mobility, strength, cardio and some type of fun factor to keep you engaged. If you follow these guidelines, your health is guaranteed to improve. It really is this simple.

Game Changing Moves:

1. Write down your goals 2x a day. One time in the morning and one time at night.
2. D.E.S. Ask yourself before every meal, "Will this help me or hurt me in achieving my goals?"
3. Workout for at least 30 minutes a day. Pick a workout that you enjoy. You will stick with what you enjoy most.

(Please use this space below)

_____

_____

_____

_____

_____

_____

_____

_____

_____

_____

"Your software controls your hardware."

#ElevatetoGreat

@CoachBrianNunez

Chapter 15

How to Choose a Mentor

Now more than ever I hear people talking all the time about how they need a mentor. Most successful people say stuff like, "You need a mentor." But they typically don't say, "Let me show you how to choose a mentor." Or, "Let me be your mentor."

But if you want to take it to the next level, you have to surround yourself with people who are already there. The blind should not lead the blind. This is the most basic criterion you can have when you are seeking to find the right mentor: they must be someone you aspire to be like.

It might be difficult for you to find that person. Maybe you aren't 100% sure about what you want to achieve, and you therefore don't know exactly who you should ask for help.

In that case, you should look at the impact that someone has made, and ask yourself if you would like to make that same sort of impact yourself. This doesn't mean you're going to become a carbon copy of that person, but it will help you decide if a potential mentor aligns with your core values or not.

For example, I don't want to be Tony Robbins, but I love the way he connects with people on stage. I don't want to be Grant Cardone, but I love the way he communicates in such a direct way. I enjoy different aspects of the way these guys teach and do things, but my goal is not to become them.

If you want to have a mentor, then the number one prerequisite you have to have is courage. This is because if you're stretching yourself and seeing a mentor who is really going to help you, then you're going to be asked to do new things, things you might not have ever done.

The first mentor I ever had was my high school football coach—Coach Lance. I went to him, and I told him that I wanted him to mentor me. His response was, "Okay, good. I just have one rule."

I was excited. I was ready to hear his million-dollar rule. What he said was, "If you ever don't do what I tell you to do, don't ever come back to me again because you're wasting my time."

In some sense, I was disappointed with this answer because I thought whatever he was going to tell me was going to be big, and this didn't seem that important at the time. But now I can see the wisdom in his words, because if I didn't listen to what he told me back then, I would not have grown by having him mentor me.

Coach Lance had a big heart, and he had a lot of compassion for people. He wanted to make an impact on a lot of kids. And he couldn't do that if when somebody came to him to be mentored, they didn't respect his time.

You respect a mentor's time by doing what they tell you to do. If you constantly question a mentor, then you're not getting value from them. If they are a good fit to be your mentor, then you should have already established that you trust their advice before becoming their mentee.

If you're not willing to listen to the answer and implement the action you're asked to implement, you're wasting not only your mentor's time, but also your own. You can learn a lot of from other people. You can be extremely engaged with the right people, but if you don't execute, nothing is going to change in your life.

My job as a mentor and coach is not to babysit the people I work with every day. I have to remind myself of this often. My job is to stretch people and push them further than they would push themselves. I learned this from Coach Lance in high school, and I've carried it with me ever since.

Everything comes back to personal responsibility. As a mentor, I help people win, but they have to do the work. Sometimes people ask questions, and they're looking for an answer. But a great mentor will help you discover the answer within yourself. Because when you can answer the question yourself, then you'll have the conviction and the courage necessary to inspire you to take action and make a move.

Great mentors are not narcissists. Narcissists only create followers. Great mentors create leaders. Great mentors are people who listen, learn and lead by example. They typically lead by questioning you and letting you develop an answer.

Bad mentors are ego driven. All they do is penalize and punish you for your mistakes. I've had more bad coaches than I've had good coaches in my life. Some of my coaches have had incredible accolades, but that doesn't mean they were great mentors. They weren't focused on the right things.

Grant Cardone says, "The pros focus on potential, and the amateurs focus on the past." A great mentor focuses on your potential. They must be a servant leader who wants to give you more than what they ask from you. Great mentors demand your best because they believe in you even when you're the most scared, not because they want you to see you struggle, even though struggle is a part of any growth process.

The temptation when choosing a mentor is to look at somebody who has everything you want, and to think that they got to where they are by taking the easy path. Everyone sees the end result of something someone has achieved, but they don't see the nightmare of what it took to achieve it.

I don't claim to be the perfect coach, but I am someone who has gone through the nightmare and came out on the other side better for it. That's why I've included all of the stories of what brought me to where I am now in this book.

We all have a past. We all have challenges we must overcome and roots we must dig out in order to live better lives. But I hope my stories and lessons have inspired you to elevate your life to the next level so you can live a more fit, focused and free lifestyle. If there's anything at all I can do to help you reach your goals, whether that be as a mentor in business or in health, don't hesitate to reach out to me.

Chapter Fifteen

Lesson

"Leaders Ask for Help"

In order to take your life or business to the next level, you have to learn from and surround yourself with people who are already there. The most important thing you have to look for when you're looking for a mentor is someone who has made the kind of impact that you want to make. You don't have to become a carbon copy of your mentor, but their values should align with yours. You have to have courage when working with a mentor, because a good one will ask you to do things that you have never done before. You must trust your mentor and do what you're asked to do, otherwise you are wasting both your time and your mentor's time. A great mentor will focus on your potential instead of your past, and they will stretch you far beyond your comfort zone.

Everyone can see the end result of something that someone has achieved, but they don't always see the nightmare it took to achieve it. Having a strong mentor will help you avoid the pitfalls that they have faced in their journey, and this will save you a lot of time, money and energy as you go through your own journey.

Every growth process requires struggle, but it's through this process that you can elevate your life to the next level. This is one of the biggest reasons to invest in a mentor or program: to learn what you don't know that you don't know. This is when growth happens and you're able to make game changing moves much faster on your way to elevating to greatness!

There is nothing I want more than for you to succeed in your life and for you to live it by your own scoreboard, set of rules and game plan. I look forward to hearing about your success living your most fit, focused and free life.

Game Changing Moves:

1. Find the people who have created the impact that you aspire to create as well. One for each category— health, wealth, relationships, and community.
2. Consume all of their content.
3. Take action based on what you have learned.
4. Personally reach out to them, expressing gratitude for their teachings.

(Please use the space below)

_____

_____

_____

_____

_____

_____

_____

_____

"If you're not willing to listen to the answer and implement the action you're asked to implement, you're wasting not only your mentor's time, but also your own."

#ElevatetoGreat
@CoachBrianNunez

Conclusion

There is no better time to take charge of your life than right now. When it comes to living your most fit, focused and free life, we need a navigation system guiding us throughout the journey. Just like you have a GPS for your car to help get you to your desired location, you need a GPS for your life. You need your own personal GPS system that will guide you and navigate you through life with more clarity, passion, purpose, conviction, courage and consistency! There is no point wasting time trying to figure out life on the fly. When you know who are, what matters most to you, and how you want to live your life, you are on the right path to living free.

You deserve you to be happy, healthy, and free. It will require hard work, sacrifice, dedication and commitment, but I guarantee you that the results of living life on your own terms will be the greatest feeling you will ever experience. There are no materialistic things that compare to the feeling of owning, sharing and embracing who you are with zero justification to anyone else.

I encourage you to start today. Use the lessons and game changing actions to write your own story for your life. Take charge and take massive action. Life is too short to not be happy and having to live life by other people's terms. You define success and create your own scoreboard. To do so, you must re-write your own rules and create new standards, not only for yourself, but for anyone else whom you choose to have in your life. Go out and create your own destiny.

YOU GET ONE LIFE TO LIVE!

Live fit. Live focused. Live FREE!

"Greatness starts with an intention to BE GREAT. There are no transitions in life, only ELEVATIONS!"

#ElevatetoGreat

@CoachBrianNunez

Thank you for reading my book.
Let's stay in touch.
I would love to support you!

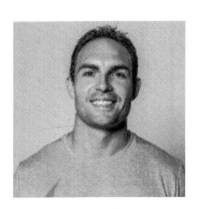

Message me on

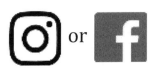 or

@CoachBrianNunez

Email
Brian@BrianNunez.com